Near Visual Acuity Tests

and Professional Vision Testing Charts

Near Visual Acuity Tests
and Professional Vision Testing Charts

by

Matthias Sachsenweger

Doctor of Medicine, Karl Marx University, Leipzig

Translated from the German by
Dr. phil. Gerhard Alexander, Leipzig

1987

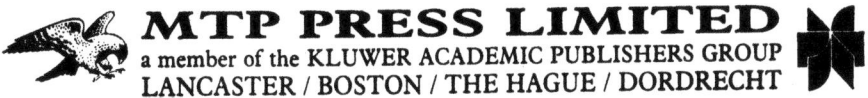

MTP PRESS LIMITED
a member of the KLUWER ACADEMIC PUBLISHERS GROUP
LANCASTER / BOSTON / THE HAGUE / DORDRECHT

Published in the UK and Europe by
MTP Press Limited
Falcon House
Lancaster, England

British Library Cataloguing in Publication Data
Sachsenweger, M.
 Near visual acuity tests and professional
 vision testing charts.
 1. Vision — Testing
 I. Title   II. Nahsehproben und
 ergophthalmologische Sehtests. *English*
 617.7'5   RE75

Published in the USA by
MTP Press
A division of Kluwer Academic Publishers
101 Philip Drive
Norwell, MA 02061, USA

Library of Congress Cataloging-in-Publication Data

Sachsenweger, Matthias.
 Near visual acuity tests and professional
vision testing charts.
 Translation of: Nahsehproben und ergophthalmologische
Sehtests.
 1. Myopia — Diagnosis. Vision — Testing. I. Title.
[DNLM: 1. Myopia — diagnosis. 2. Vision Tests — instrumentation. WW 320 S 121n]
RE938.S2313   1986   617.7'55   86-27363

ISBN 978-90-481-5801-0

Copyright © 1987 MTP Press Limited
Softcover reprint of the hardcover 1st edition 1987

All rights reserved. No part of this publication
may be reproduced, stored in a retrieval
system, or transmitted in any form or by any
means, electronic, mechanical, photocopying,
recording or otherwise, without permission
from the publishers.

Preface

In the last decade the field of occupational medicine within ophthalmology (ergophthalmology) has advanced remarkably not only by the intensive activities of several ophthalmologists but also as a consequence of the increasing importance of visual problems in the world of work, especially with regard to rehabilitation, determination of ability, prevention of impairment of vision etc. As a result of this there is an immense deficiency of suitable test methods relevant to practice in the form of short-distance vision testing charts. It is true, in the majority of cases, that the usual vision tests are also sufficient for questions of occupational medicine; these can often be replaced partly by specific tests. Nevertheless, many physicians will regard it as advantageous, when, apart from the usual reading texts, they can also demonstrate to their patients examples for particular visual requirements in daily life and in various professions.

The following short-distance vision testing charts fulfil this task. They are regarded as a beginning. The number of tests might easily be increased under the various categories. The reading texts have been put together with different printing types from newspapers and books, always with an indication to which of the usual short-distance vision tests they correspond. The test distance should always be noted in the documentation of the test result.

In order to prevent too rapid wear when the test charts are frequently used an additional test type for everyday use is enclosed which can be preserved in a clear cover, if necessary. The patterns for the screen reading device and the braille serve for rehabilitative purposes.
I hope that these charts prove useful in daily practice.

Matthias Sachsenweger

Contents

Unspecific tests

test 1	Landolt's rings	8–13
test 2	Numbers	14–18
test 3	Pflueger's hooks	19–23
test 4	Reading tests	24–27
test 5	Reading tests in French and German	28–29
test 6	Different type-writer characters	30
test 7	Printed letters for amblyopes	31
test 8	Handoptotypes	32–33
test 9	Vernier acuity I	34–35
test 10	Vernier acuity II	34–35
test 11		36–37
test 12	Other vision testing charts	36–37
test 13		36–37

Typical test types for special professions

test 14	Groups of lines	38
test 15	Pencil-line calibres (gradation degrees)	39
test 16	Caliper (for calibre and lumen measurements)	40
test 17	Tape measure	40
test 18	Slide-rule	41
test 19	Protractor	41
test 20	Graphs	42
test 21	Technical microscopy	42
test 22	Medical microscopy	43
test 23	Chemical formula	44
test 24	Mathematical formula	44
test 25	Circuit diagram	45

test 26	Punched tape for electronic data processing	46
test 27	Punched card for electronic data processing	46
test 28	Aerialphotograph (scale 1:6000)	47
test 29	Aerialphotograph (scale 1:12500)	47
test 30	Plan of a city	48
test 31	Map I	49
test 32	Map II	49
test 33	Notes – visual testing charts I	50–51
test 34	Notes – visual testing charts II	50–52

Everyday tests

test 35	Part of the telephone directory	53
test 36	Newspaper types	53
test 37	Tickets	54
test 38	Time-table	55

Test types for special purposes

test 39	Vision testing charts for the screen reading device	
test 40	(positive and negative picture reproduction)	55–57
test 41	Anaglyph	58–59
test 42	Examination of the central visual field	60
test 43	Measurement of short-distance exo- and esophoria	61
test 44	Braille	
test 45	Relief demonstration for the blind	

Literature	62

Additional test type for everyday use

Unspecific tests / d = 1 m

TESTS 1-3

TEST 1   Landolt's rings

TEST 2   Numbers

TEST 3   Pflueger's hooks

In every test line the visual acuity (= V) is recorded. This is necessary for the recognition of optotypes at a test distance of 1 m. A conversion for other test distances is easily possible. The size of the individual optotypes, their relation to Landolt's ring as well as their gradation depend on international propositions.

Unspecific tests / d = 1 m

TEST 1

V = 2,0

V = 1,6

V = 1,25

V = 1,0

V = 0,8

V = 0,63

V = 0,5

V = 0,4

V = 0,32

V = 0,25

V = 0,2

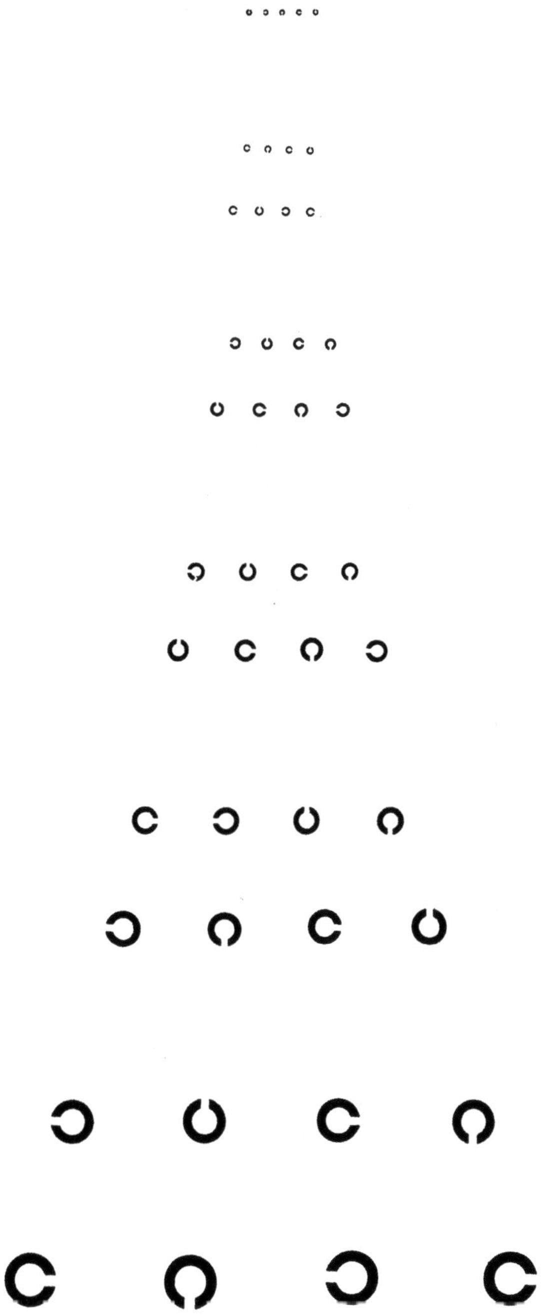

Unspecific tests / d = 1 m

TEST 1

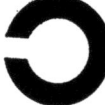

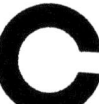

V = 0,16   V = 0,1

Unspecific tests / d = 1 m

TEST 1

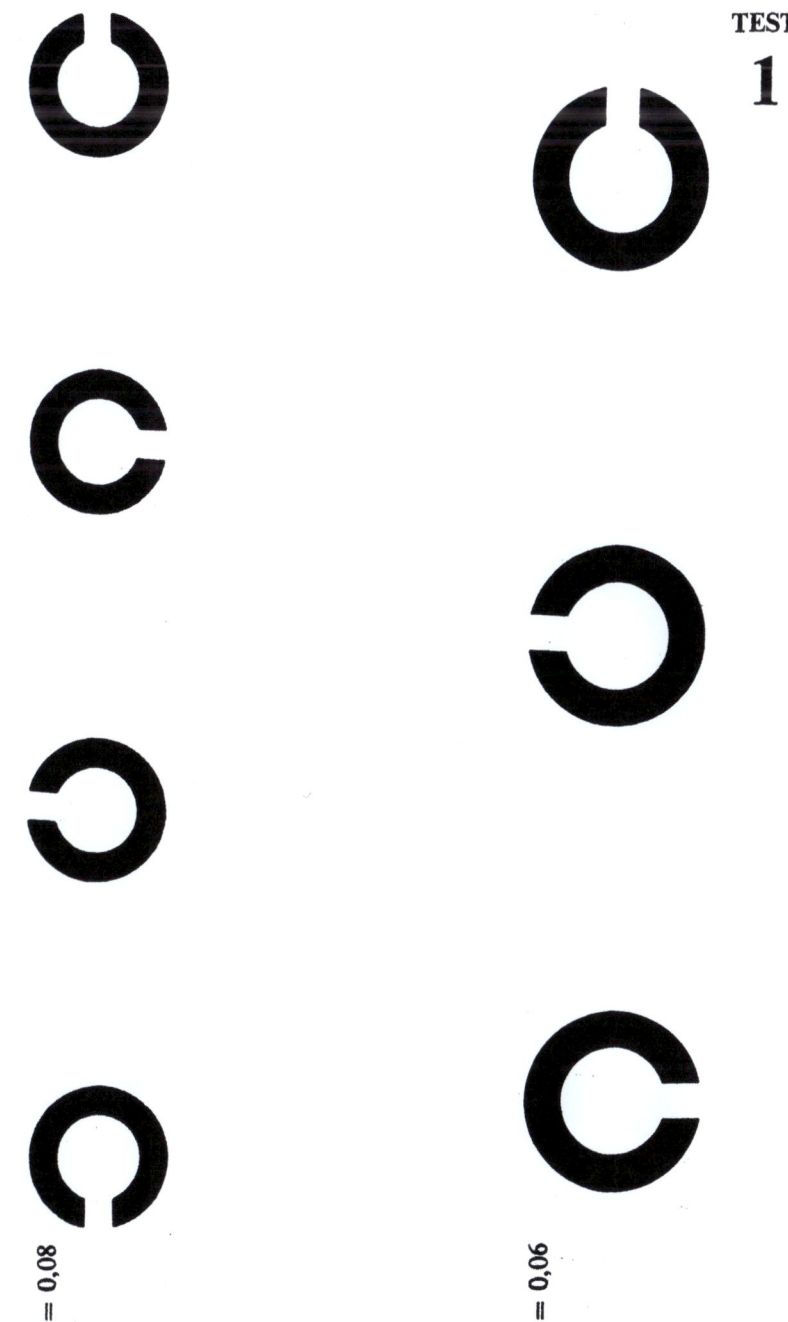

V = 0,08

V = 0,06

Unspecific tests / d = 1 m 12

TEST 1

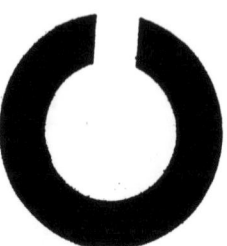
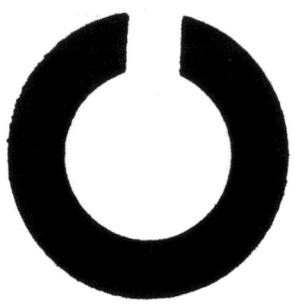
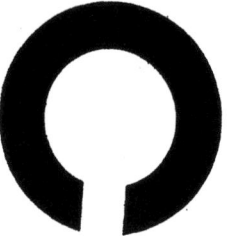
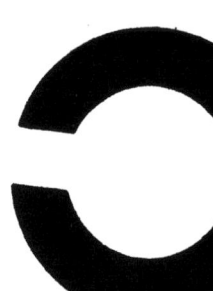
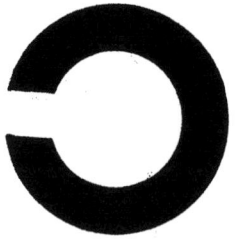

V = 0,05

V = 0,04

Unspecific tests / d = 1 m

TEST 1

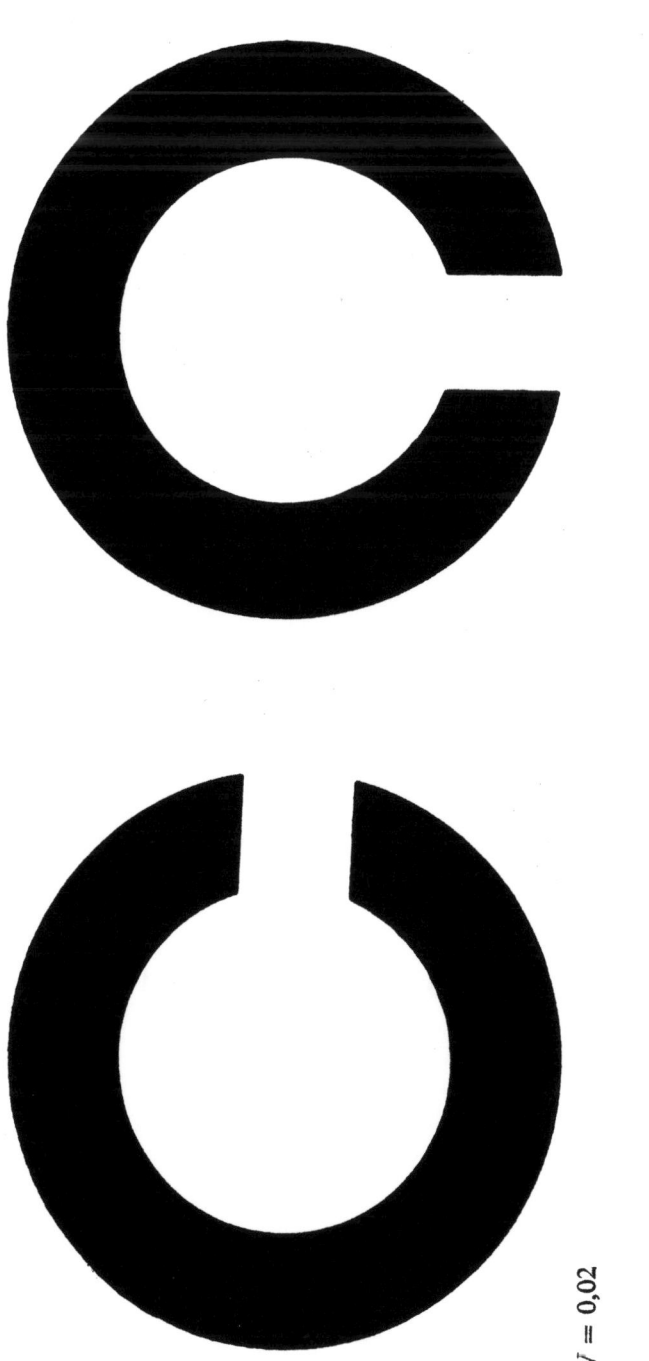

V = 0,02

TEST 2

3 2 0 9	V = 2,0
6 7 2 0 6	V = 1,6
9 6 0 2 7	V = 1,25
6 0 2 3	V = 1,0
2 0 3 4	V = 0,8
2 0 4 3	V = 0,63
6 7 9 4	V = 0,5
3 4 7 6	V = 0,4
3 2 0 4	V = 0,32
0 2 3 6	V = 0,25
3 4 9 2	V = 0,2

TEST
2

V = 0,16 9 4 6 7

V = 0,1 7 3 6 4

Unspecific tests / d = 1 m 16

TEST 2

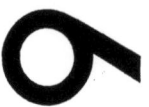
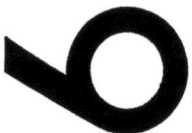
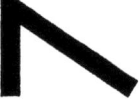
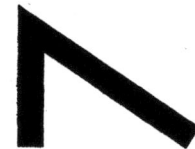
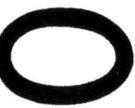
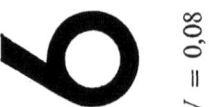
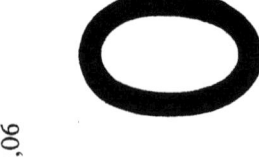

V = 0,08

V = 0,06

Unspecific tests / d = 1 m

TEST 2

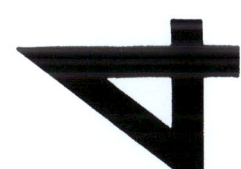
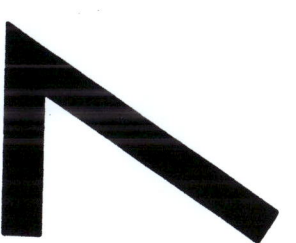

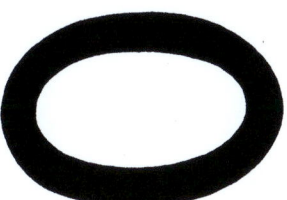
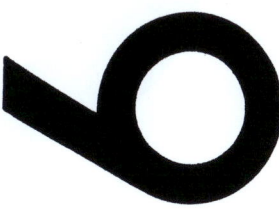

V = 0,05
V = 0,04

Unspecific tests / d = 1 m

TEST 2

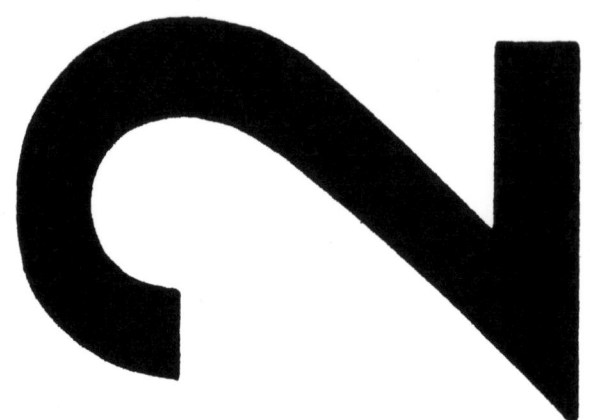

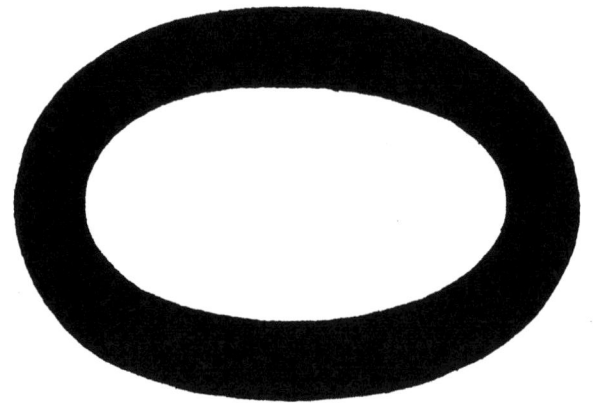

V = 0,02

Unspezific tests / d = 1m

TEST 3

V = 2,0

V = 1,6
V = 1,25

V = 1,0
V = 0,8

V = 0,63
V = 0,5

V = 0,4

V = 0,32

V = 0,25

V = 0,2

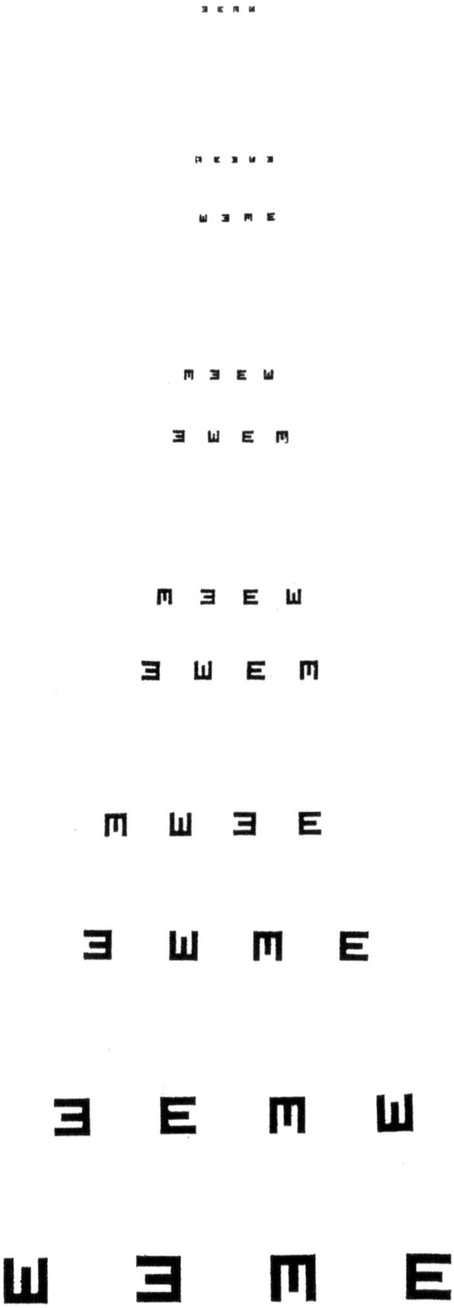

Unspezific tests / d = 1 m 20

TEST 3

E
E
Ǝ
ω
E

E
E
Ǝ
ω

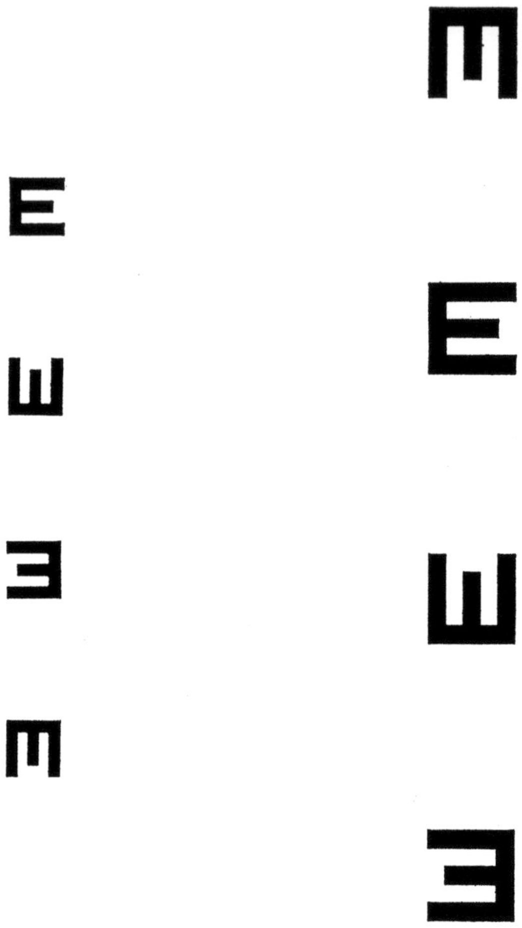

V = 0,16

V = 0,1

Unspecific tests / d = 1 m

TEST 3

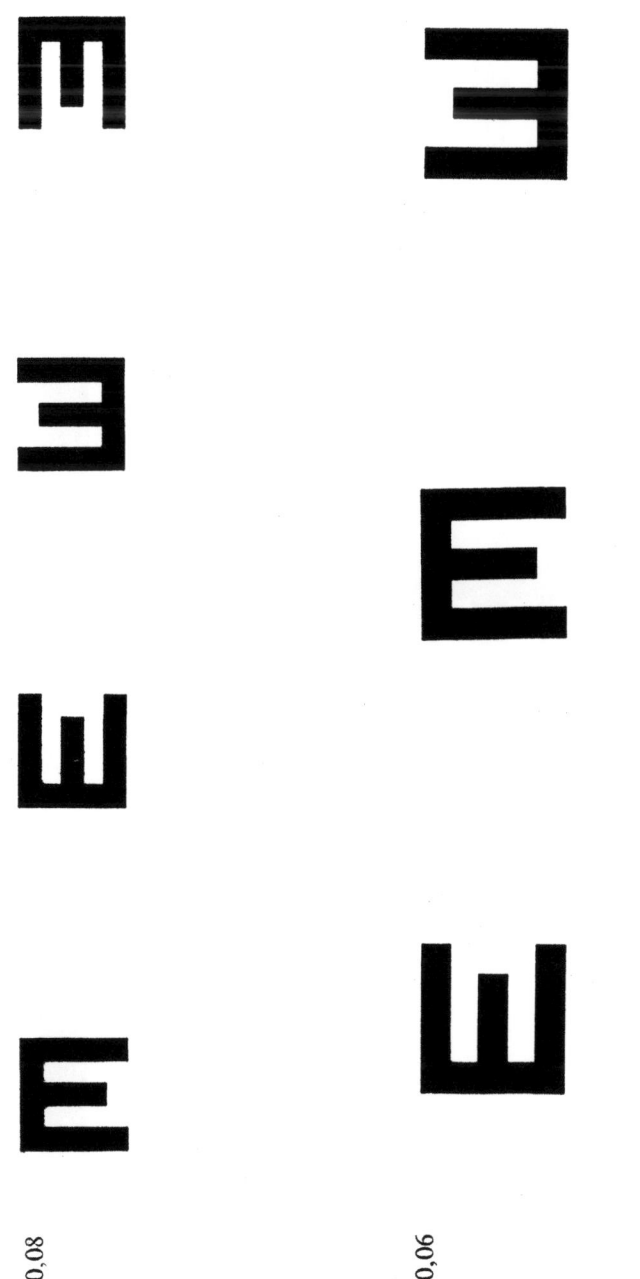

V = 0,08

V = 0,06

Unspecific tests / d = 1 m   22

TEST 3

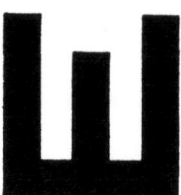

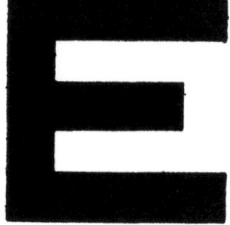

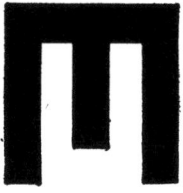

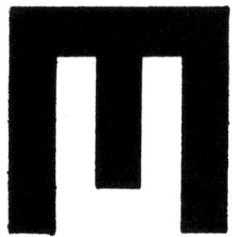

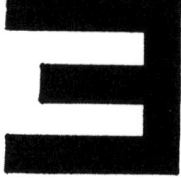

V = 0,05   V = 0,04

23 Unspecific tests / d = 1 m

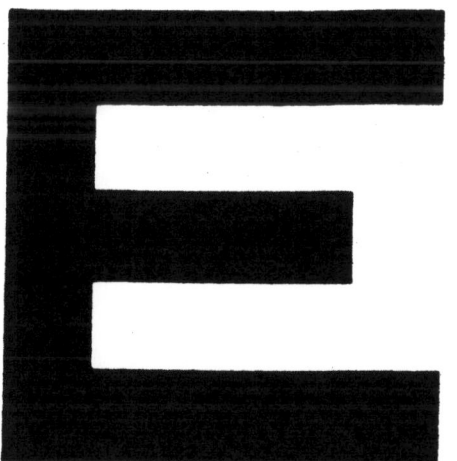

TEST
3

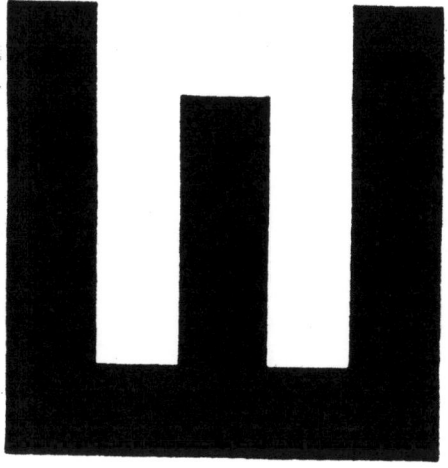

V = 0,02

TEST **Reading tests**

The test 4 contains short-distance reading tests in various types, which are common in newspaper and book printing (Univers medium, Times medium, Univers bold, Times italic) and in different sizes with particulars of size in the internationally valid printers' "point" system (N). In addition, above these details adequate vision is noted in decimals for an observation distance of 30 cm. Larger types (N. = 18, N. = 20, N. = 28, N. = 36, N. = 42, N. = 48 and N. = 60) are printed in Univers medium.

Conversion of the sizes of types in decimals, fraction, and other reading tests

typographic measuring system (N.)	adequate vision (d = 30 cm)	vision in fraction	other reading tests		
			Nieden	Snellen	Jaeger
N. 3	1.0	0.3/0.3	–	1	1
N. 4	0.75	0.3/0.4	1	1.5	2
N. 5	0.6	0.3/0.5	2	2	3
N. 6	0.5	0.3/0.6	3	2.5	4
N. 7	0.43	0.3/0.7	4	3	5
N. 8	0.38	0.3/0.8	5	–	6
N. 9	0.33	0.3/0.9	6	3.5	8
N. 10	0.3	0.3/1.0	–	–	–
N. 11	0.27	0.3/1.1	7	4	9
N. 12	0.25	0.3/1.2	8	4.5	10
N. 14	0.21	0.3/1.4	–	–	–
N. 16	0.19	0.3/1.6	–	5	11
N. 18	0.17	0.3/1.8	9	5.5	12
N. 20	0.15	0.3/2.0	–	6	13
N. 24	0.13	0.3/2.4	10	7.5	14
N. 28	0.11	0.3/2.8	–	9	15
N. 36	0.08	0.3/3.6	11	12	16
N. 42	0.07	0.3/4.2	–	13.5	–
N. 48	0.06	0.3/4.8	12	15	17
N. 60	0.05	0.3/6.0	13	–	–

N. 3 / V = 1.0

The Gulf Stream comes from the Gulf of Mexico and brings warm water to the coasts of Western Europe. – 3 78 364 4567 87534 198034 1763458 99586712 109458356 1856403684 87453827109 7453821095346

The Panama Canal, an artificial water way, connects the Pacific with the Atlantic Ocean. – 3 75 345 6143

The Atlas Mountains in North Africa lead from the Atlantic Ocean along the coast of the Mediterranean Sea to the Gulf of Tunisia. – 6 26 364 2923 46612 364123 3082164 19584734 194867324 10857483673

The Straits of Gibraltar are a connection between the Mediterranean Sea and the Atlantic Ocean. – 3 75 175 3432

N. 4 / V = 0.75

The Sahara in North Africa, the largest desert of the world, comprises about 7 to 9 million square kilometres. – 7 34 357 9871 21238 091328 7832109 12345678

The difference in altitude between Lake Erie and Lake Ontario is spanned by the Niagara Falls. – 2 96 543 1234 54678 909876 5432123 45678909 876543212

The Cheviot Hills are the border mountains between England and Scotland. – 2 88 123 4567 89098 765432 3573412 34567896 0765432123 19846673210

The Caucasus is a system of fold-mountains between the Black Sea and the Caspian Sea. – 6 87 936 4589 86417

N. 5 / V = 0.6

Mount Vesuvius, south-east of Naples, is the only active volcano of the European continent. – 3 75 123 3454 12345 678909

The Amazon is considered to be the largest river of South America and the most abounding in water of the entire Earth. – 7 38

Lake Victoria, the largest lake of Africa, is located 1134 m above sea-level. – 6 90 876 5432 12345 678909 1435687 23456098

The Baltic Sea is an inland sea between Central, North and North-East Europe. – 1 87 123 4567 89012 742509 1658790 543212345

N. 6 / V = 0.5

The Andes extend along the west coast of the South American continent. – 6 58 670 6521 5824930

The Cambrian Mountains occupy a large part of the peninsula of Wales. – 6 49 824 6019 473428 7654321

The highland of Tibet is located on average 4000 to 5000 m above sea-level. – 3 57 840 6125 7048523

Indonesia is an archipelago between Asia and Australia. 9 86 765 3124 97341

N. 7 / V = 0.43

The Ural Mountains and the River Ural form the boundary between Europe and Asia. – 9

The Bosporus is crossed by a bridge.
5 61 234 8716 95312

The highest and most spectacular fold-mountains of the earth are the Himalaya Mountains. – 8 17 653 4902 45286 675409 456

The Alps are the highest and most extensive mountains of Europe. – 3 45 396 6518 87463 2389546

N. 8 / V = 0.38

On Iceland there are numerous active volcanos. – 8 45 790 2356 09876 123456

The Elbrooz is, at 5633 m, the highest mountain in the Caucasus. – 1 23 4567

The coast of the Crimean Peninsula is washed by the Black Sea and the Sea of Azov. – 7 56 465 9023 58734 1234567

The Dardanelles connect the Black Sea with the Mediterranean Sea. – 9 34 6023 27909

N. 9 / V = 0.33

Australia is considered to be the smallest continent. – 1 56 768 9876

Cape Horn is the southernmost point of South America. – 9 26 714 6580

The Caspian Sea is the largest lake in the world. – 7 256 9342

The Red Sea has a length of more than 2300 km. – 4 82 376 9012 45372

Unspecific tests / d = 30 cm

N. 10 / V = 0.3

The Indian Ocean is the smallest of the three oceans. – 6 35

The Nile is, at 6671 km, the longest river of the earth. – 5 67 201

Rotterdam possesses the largest seaport of Europe. – 3 247

Greenland is considered to be the largest island in the world. – 1 468

N. 11 / V = 0.27

The Volga is considered to be the longest river of Europe. – 7 45 908 2156 34897 145

The length of the Danube is 2860 km. – 6 25 207 4569

The capital of Hungary is Budapest. – 3 87 968 2057

The Isle of Man is located in the Irish Sea. – 9 85 274 8307 98

N. 12 / V = 0.25

Berne is the capital of Switzerland. – 3 68 4708

Venice is built on 107 islands. – 2 67 482 7903 09

The Mississippi is the largest river of North America. – 7 23 856 0987

Brazil is the largest country of Latin America. – 3 74 905

N. 14 / V = 0.21

Odessa is on the Black Sea. – 5 80 641 7325

Highland of Iran.
5 34 961 8945 31258

Sicily is in the Mediterranean Sea. – 6 49 408

*Scandinavian peninsula.
2 54 687 9431 86597*

N. 16 / V = 0.19

Frankfurt-on-Main. – 3 48 625

The Persian Gulf.
6 82 125 8969 54138

**Shetland Islands.
6 81 735 9804 67413**

*Stratford-upon-Avon.
9 52 967 4531 89451*

Unspecific tests / d = 30 cm

N. 18 / V = 0.17

The Highlands of Scotland. — 8 64 275

N. 20 / V = 0.15

Vienna on the Danube. — 9 32 785

N. 24 / V = 0.13

Great Britain. — 1 563 12 7903

N. 28 / V = 0.11

Pacific Ocean. — 4 78 9034

N. 36 / V = 0.08

Amsterdam. — 7 643

N. 42 / V = 0.07

North Sea. — 5 86

N. 48 / V = 0.06

Africa. — 8 54 5

N. 60 / V = 0.05

London. — 7

Unspecific tests / d = 30 cm

TEST
5
Reading tests in French and German

N. 3 / V = 1.0

Le Rhône qui prend sa source dans les Alpes de Berne, est le plus abondant des fleuves français. − 7 38

Der Grosse Inselsberg, eine Erhebung des Thüringer Waldes, liegt unmittelbar auf dem Rennsteig. − 6

N. 4 / V = 0.75

Le lac Leman se trouve à 372 mètres au-dessus de la mer et a une profondeur de 309 mètres. − 8 17 653 8407 29431 294765 0987654 13246587 019283756 123

Der Loreleifelsen ragt 132 m über den Rhein empor, der an dieser Stelle 113 m breit ist. − 0 98 765 4321 09876 543212 3456789 13245670 927645120 012343

N. 5 / V = 0.6

La Normandie est située de part et d'autre de la basse Seine au nord de la France. − 6 85 760 5216 67450 760521 0987654

In der Nähe von Innsbruck am Fuße des Karwendelgebirges liegt der 750 m hohe Berg Isel. − 1 23 456 7890 98765 432123

N. 6 / V = 0.5

Le pas de Calais a une largeur de 31 km à son point le plus étroit. − 5 37 480 2561 40725 368470 1234567

An den Bodensee grenzen die Schweiz, Österreich und die Bundesrepublik Deutschland. − 5 37 480

N. 7 / V = 0.43

Le Pyrénées constituent la frontière entre la France et l'Espagne. − 3 26 709 5632 12875

Rostock befindet sich 12 km von der Mündung der Warnow in die Ostsee entfernt. − 3

N. 8 / V = 0.38

Le mont Blanc est le sommet le plus élevé de l'Europe. − 2 69 805 7246 1574

Heidelberg liegt am Eintritt des Neckars in die Rheinebene. − 2 69 805 7246 15749

N. 9 / V = 0.33

La Corse est la plus grande île française de la Mediterranée. − 4 695

Die Nordseeinsel Helgoland ragt bis zu 56 m aus dem Meer. − 4 69

N. 10 / V = 0.3

Marseille est le premier port de commerce de France. − 5 37 879

Zürich liegt am Nordrand des Zürichsees. − 5 37 879 143213

N. 12 / V = 0.25

Monaco est situé sur la côte d'Azur. − 9 13 536 89

Wien ist die Hauptstadt Österreichs. − 9 13 536 21

N. 14 / V = 0.21

Le Mont-Saint-Michel.

Mecklenburger Seen. −

N. 16 / V = 0.19

Clermont-Ferrand. —   Frankfurt am Main —

N. 18 / V = 0.17

Le golfe du Lion. —   Erzgebirge. —613

N. 20 / V = 0.15

Cherbourg. — 9   Rheinebene.—2

N. 24 / V = 0.13

Champagne.   Matterhorn. —

N. 28 / V = 0.11

Bordeaux. —   Zugspitze. —

N. 36 / V = 0.08

Grenoble   Hamburg

N. 48 / V = 0.06

Paris. 4   Berlin 5

N. 60 / V = 0.05

Lyon.   Harz.

Unspecific tests

TEST 6   Different type-writer characters

Loch Ness is situated in the northern
Scottish valley of Glenmore.
Glasgow is the largest town of Scotland.
**Oxford and Cambridge are the oldest
university towns of Great Britain.**
The English Channel connects the North Sea with the Atlantic Ocean.
Sicily is the largest island in the Mediterranean Sea.
Three European capitals are situated on the Danube.
𝔗𝔥𝔢 𝔠𝔞𝔲𝔠𝔞𝔰𝔲𝔰 𝔦𝔰 𝔰𝔦𝔱𝔲𝔞𝔱𝔢𝔡 𝔟𝔢𝔱𝔴𝔢𝔢𝔫 𝔱𝔥𝔢 𝔅𝔩𝔞𝔠𝔨 𝔞𝔫𝔡 𝔱𝔥𝔢 ℭ𝔞𝔰𝔭𝔦𝔞𝔫 𝔖𝔢𝔞𝔰.
The island of Cuba belongs to the Great Antilles.
The North Cape is said to be the northern most point of Europe.
Los Angeles is situated on the west coast
of the United States.
Moscow is the largest town in the Soviet Union.
The Brenner Pass is the lowest pass across the Central Alps.
Dublin is the capital of the Irish Republic.

Printed letters for amblyopes　　　　　　　　　　　　TEST

Printed books for amblyopes usually contain different kinds and sizes of printing. Three examples are given.

7

The Isle of Man is located in the Irish Sea. – 432 2817 12345 678

Edinburgh is the capital of Scotland. – 493 8278

The Thames has a length of 336 km. – 593 8265 89630

Unspecific tests / d = 1 m

TEST 8 **Hand optotypes**

These serve for the orienting testing of visual acuity in pre-school children and illiterates. 1 m is the distance to the visual testing chart in this test. The patient to be tested should position his or her hand in such a way that he or she sees the black hand on the visual testing chart. After preliminary exercises two-year-old children should recognize with each eye individually the signs of the 3rd series, three-year-olds those of the 2nd series and older children those of the 1st series.

Unspecific tests / d = 1 m

TEST 8

V = 1,0 · · · · · I

V = 0,63 II

V = 0,5 III

V = 0,4

V = 0,32

V = 0,25

V = 0,2

V = 0,16

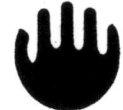 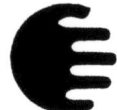 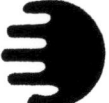 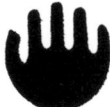

V = 0,1

Unspecific tests

TEST 9   **Vernier acuity I**

In test 9 it shall be shown whether and where the middle part of the respective lines is displaced to the right or the left. In line (a) the displacement is 1 mm to the left, in line (b) 0.75 mm to the left, in line (c) 0.5 mm to the right, in line (d) 0.4 mm to the right, in line (e) 0.3 mm to the right, in line (f) 0.2 mm to the right, in line (g) 0.1 mm to the right, in line (h) 0.08 mm to the right, and in line (i) 0.06 mm to the left.

TEST 10   **Vernier acuity II**

In test 10 the beam of the cross, the outer half of which in displaced, is to be identified. In cross (a) the displacement is 1 mm, in cross (b) and (c) 0.5 mm, in cross (d) and (e) 0.25 mm, in cross (f) and (g) 0.1 mm, in cross (h), (i) and (j) 0.06 mm.

35　　　　　　　　　　　　　　　　　　　　　　　　　　Unspecific tests

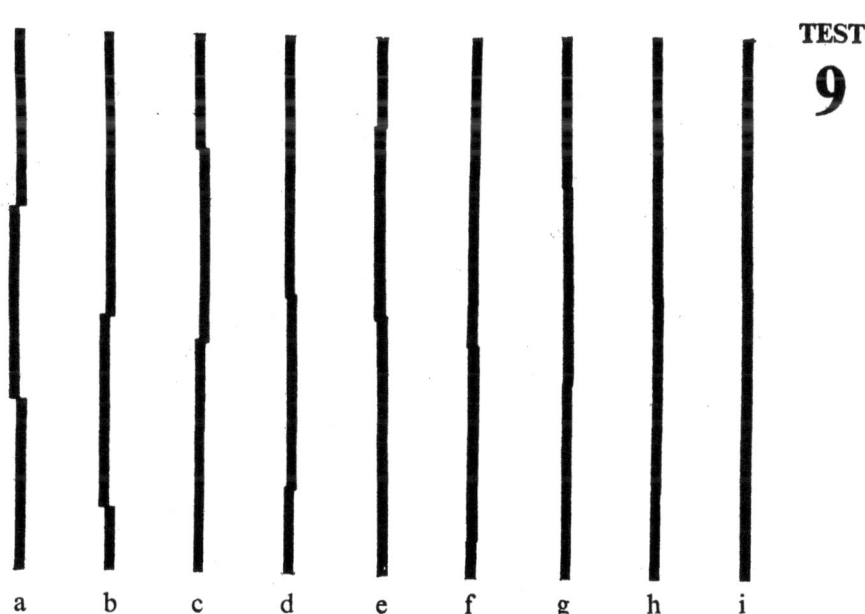

TEST 9

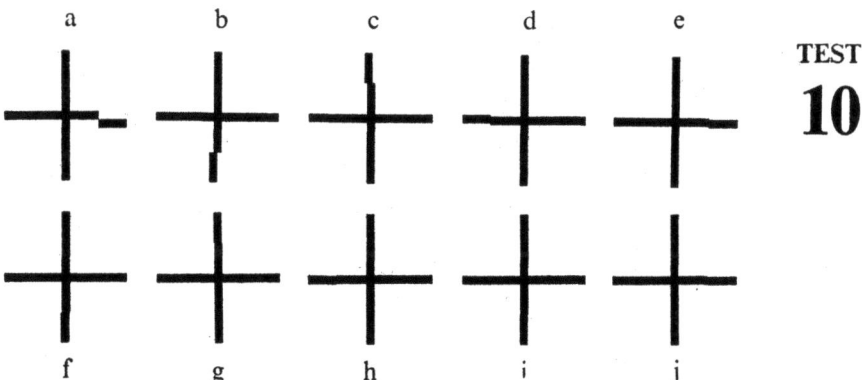

TEST 10

3*

Unspecific tests

TEST **Other vision testing charts**
11-
13

TEST
11
The patient is asked to count the squares in the middle series of the tests a to g. The length of the margins of the squares is 10 mm in test (a), 5 mm in test (b), 3 mm in test (c), 2 mm in test (d), 1 mm in test (e), 0.5 mm in test (f), 0.3 mm in test (g), and 0.2 mm in test (h).

TEST
12
The numbers of the middle series are to be read in the horizontal and the vertical directions respectively. An insufficiency of separating power is indicated when the recognizability of the numbers in the squares is worse than the adequate near vision acuity. In (a) the squares of the numbers correspond to N. 11, in (b) N. 8, in (c) N. 7, in (d) N. 6, and in (e) N. 4.

TEST
13
Among the 4 squares of a test figure 1 square has changed its form. In test (a) this square is located above, in test (b) below, in test (c) to the left, in test d to the right, in test (e) below, in test (f) above, in test (g) to the left, and in test (h) to the right.

37   **Unspecific tests**

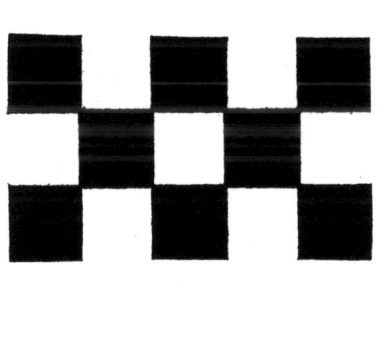

a

TEST
11

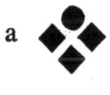 a

 b

 c

 d

 e

 f

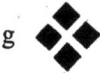 g

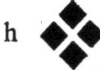 h

TEST
13

b

c

d

e
f
g
h

52497294	21675249	42759342	72945249	93452425
37723169	53093772	69837017	31693772	70123843
13654755	48531365	52412659	47551365	71453753
08412423	67420841	37537445	24230841	
a	b	c	d	e

TEST
12

Typical test types for special professions

TEST 14 **Groups of lines**

This test contains the groups of lines which are used together in technical drawing (full lines, dashed lines, dash-dot lines, free-hand lines). The thickness of the lines is given in mm.

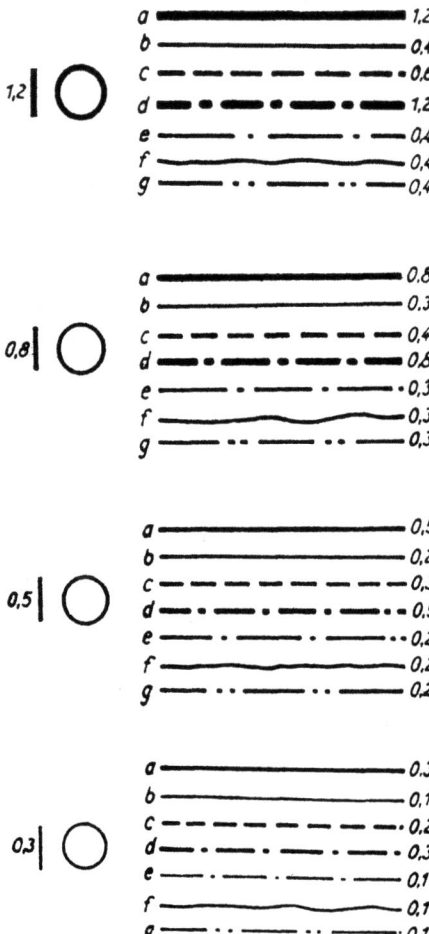

Pencil-line calibres (gradation degress)

This contains the usual calibres of pencil-lines: (a) and (b) are used commonly in office departments and at school, (c)–(e) mostly for technical drawing, and (f)–(g) mostly for lithography.

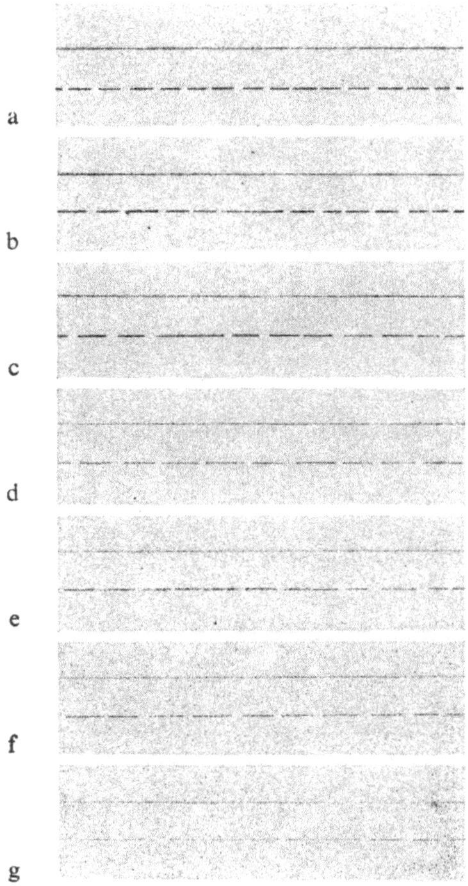

TEST
15

a

b

c

d

e

f

g

Typical test types for special professions   40

TEST 16   **Calliper** (for calibre and lumen measurements)

The question is asked which lines correspond above and below the dividing line: (a) = 5.36, (b) = 4.68, (c) = 5.09 ($\triangleq$ vernier acuity).

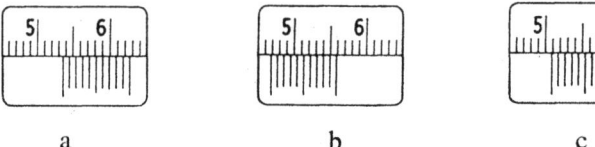

a   b   c

TEST 17   **Tape measure**

The patient is asked which values are indicated by the lines coming from above (a = 73.5; b = 86.2).

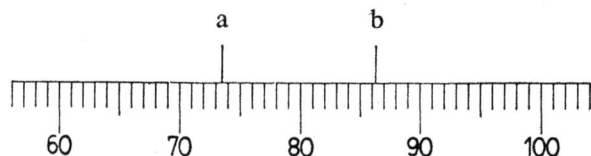

Slide-rule

TEST 18

The person tested is asked at which value the longitudinal line cuts the several scales (a–f) (a: 41.9; b: 12.05; c: 72.7; d: 42.84; e: 2.695; f: 3.475).

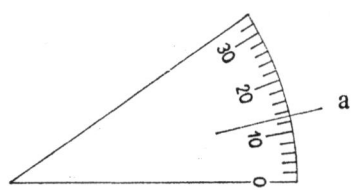

Protactor

TEST 19

The patient is asked which angle is indicated by line (a) (13°).

TEST 20 **Graphs**

The patient is asked for coordinates of some of the symbols in both diagrams.

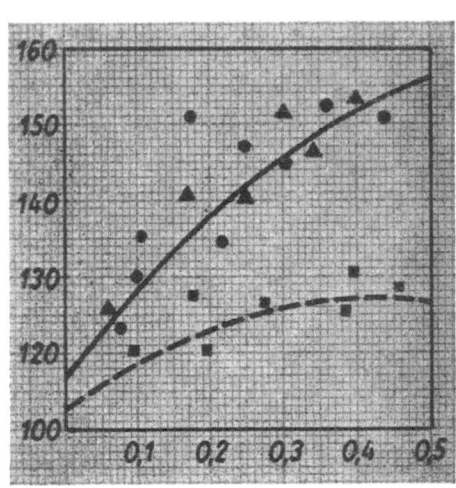
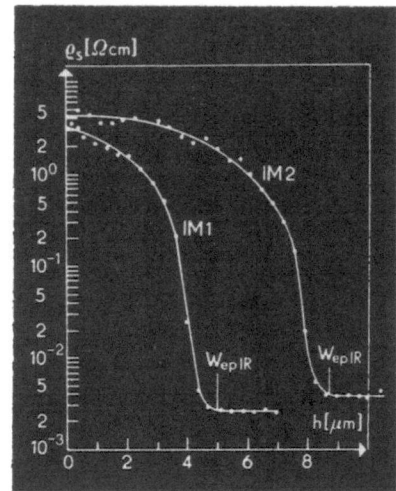

TEST 21 **Technical microscopy**

All the demonstrated details of the light-microscopic figures from mineralogy should be recognized.

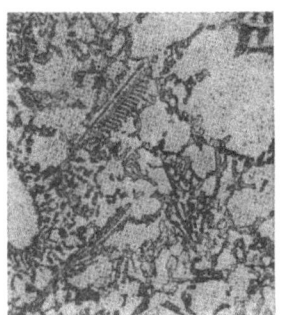
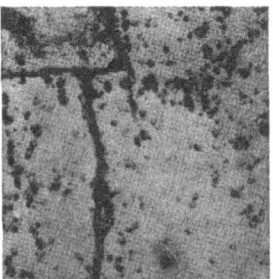
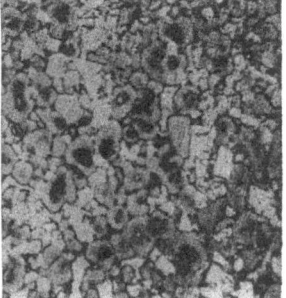

Medical microscopy

TEST 22

a) The patient is asked the number of cells (leucocytes) located within the four group squares (grids with 16 fields each).

b) In the urine sediment the various cell structures are to be described.

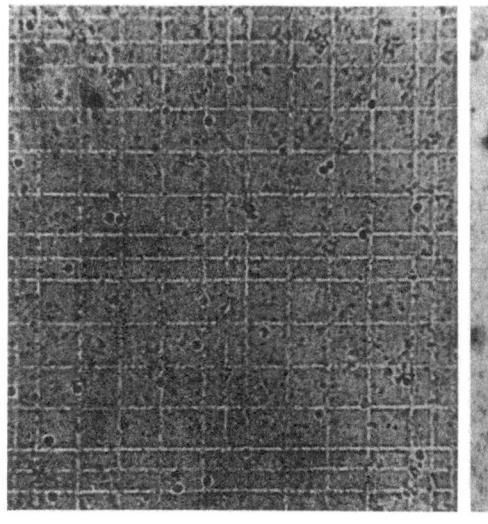
a

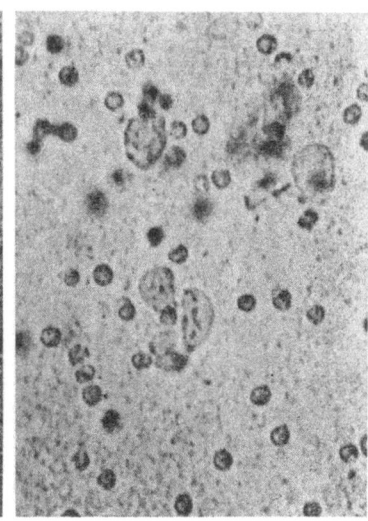
b

Typical test types for special professions

TEST   Chemical formula

23

[Structural formula of a quinone with long isoprenoid side chain: a benzoquinone ring bearing two H, and $-CH_3$, connected via $-CH_2-CH(CH_3)-CH_2-CH_2-CH(CH_3)-CH_2-CH_2-CH(CH_3)-CH_2-CH_2-CH(CH_3)-CH_3$]

[Structural formula of riboflavin: isoalloxazine ring system with H_3C- and H_3C- substituents on the benzene ring, and ribitol side chain $-CH_2-H-C-H-HO-C-H-HO-C-H-HO-C-H-CH_2OH$]

TEST   Mathematical formula

24

$$t_E = \frac{t'_E + x'_E \cdot V/c^2}{\sqrt{1 - V^2/c^2}}$$

$$t_E = \frac{1\,s - \dfrac{3 \cdot 10^8\,m \cdot 1{,}8 \cdot 10^8\,m \cdot s^{-1}}{(3 \cdot 10^8\,m \cdot s^{-1})^2}}{\sqrt{1 - \dfrac{(1{,}8 \cdot 10^8\,m \cdot s^{-1})^2}{(3 \cdot 10^8\,m \cdot s^{-1})^2}}}$$

$$t_E = \frac{1\,s - \dfrac{6}{10}\,s}{\sqrt{1 - \dfrac{36}{100}}}$$

Typical test types for special professions

Circuit diagram

TEST 25

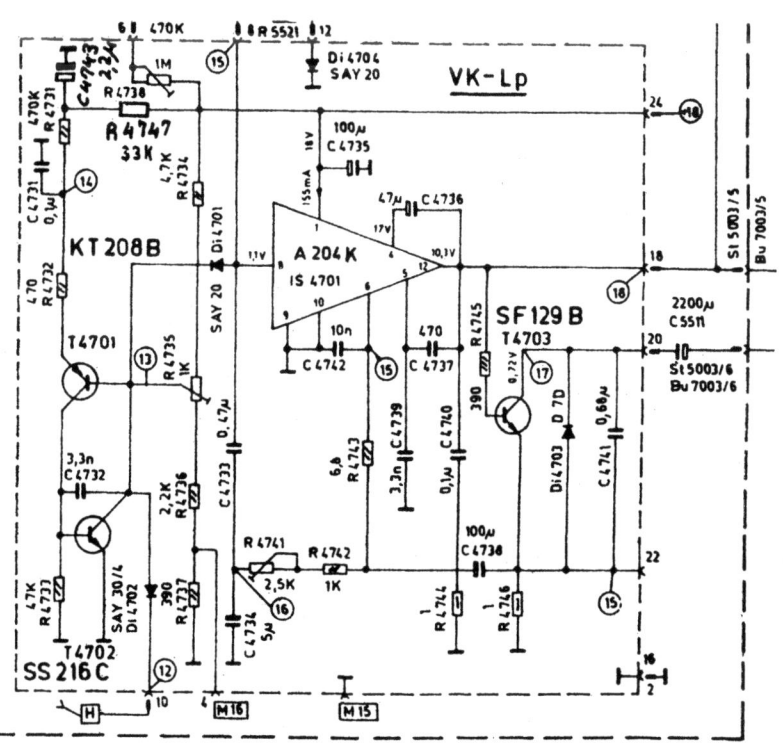

Typical test types for special professions 46

TEST 26 Punched tape for electronic data processing

TEST 27 Punched card for electronic data processing

Typical test types for special professions

Aerialphotograph (scale 1:6000)　　　　　　　　　　　TEST
28

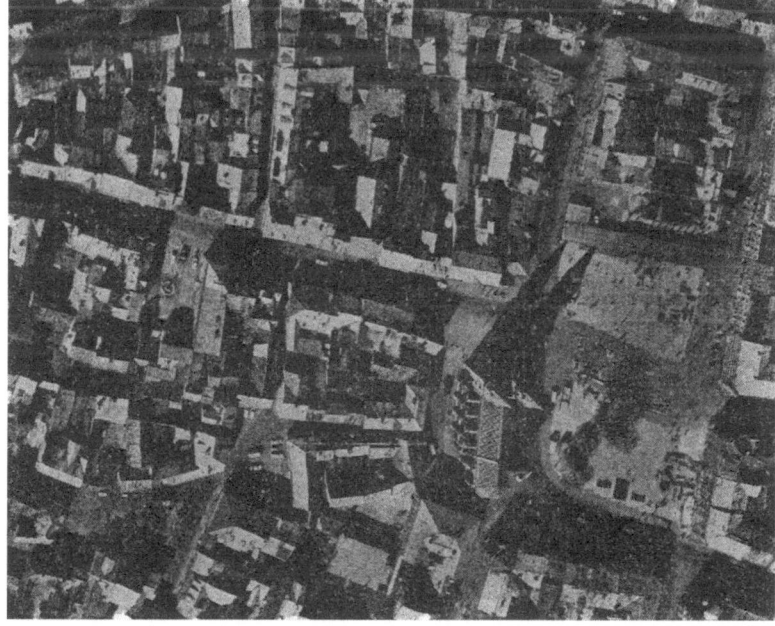

Aerialphotograph (scale 1:12500)　　　　　　　　　　TEST
29

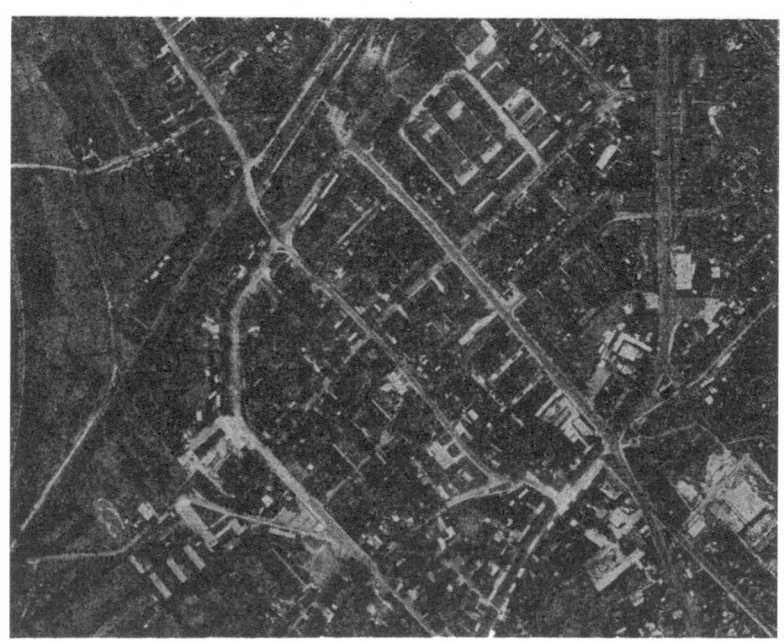

Typical test types for special professions 48

TEST 30   **Plan of a city**

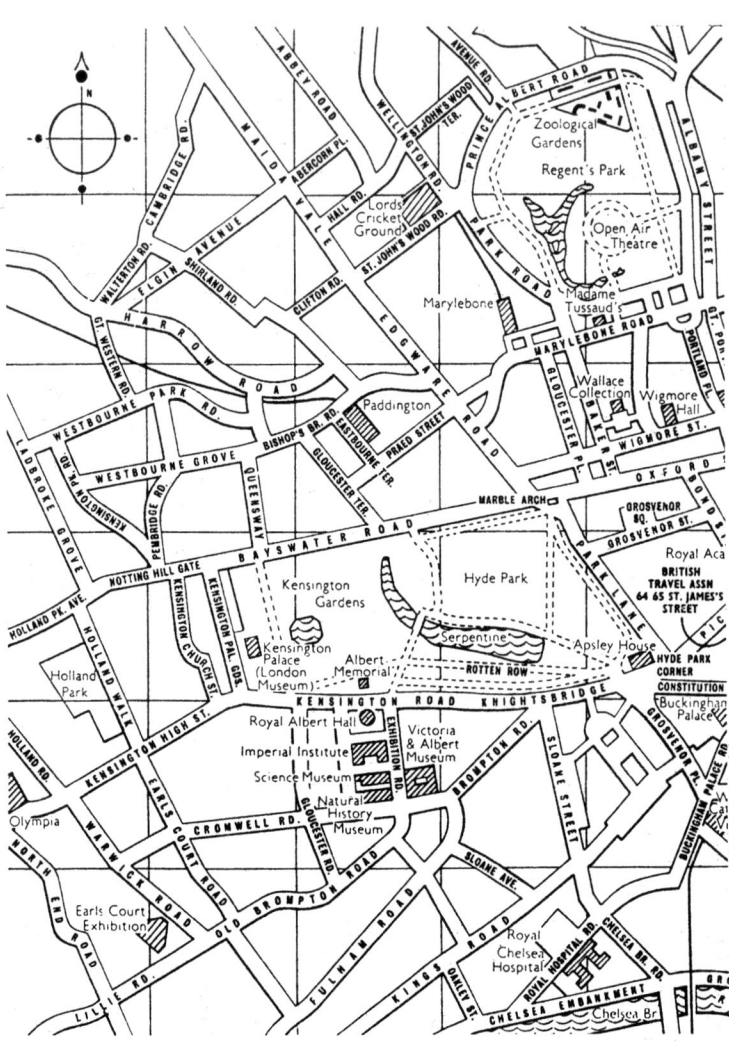

Typical test types for special professions

Map I

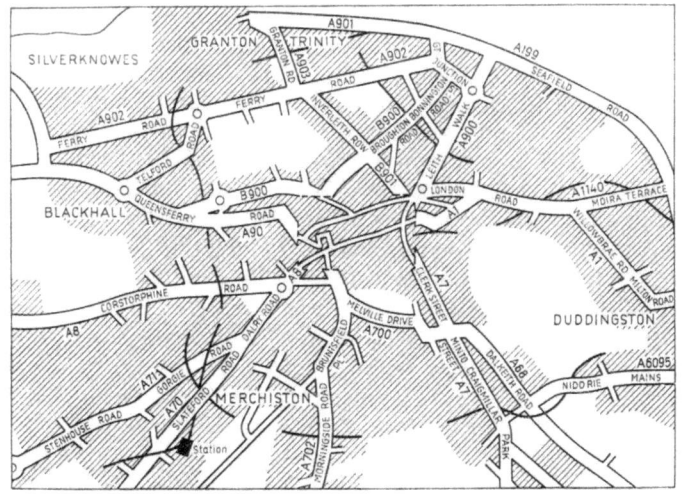

TEST
31

Map II

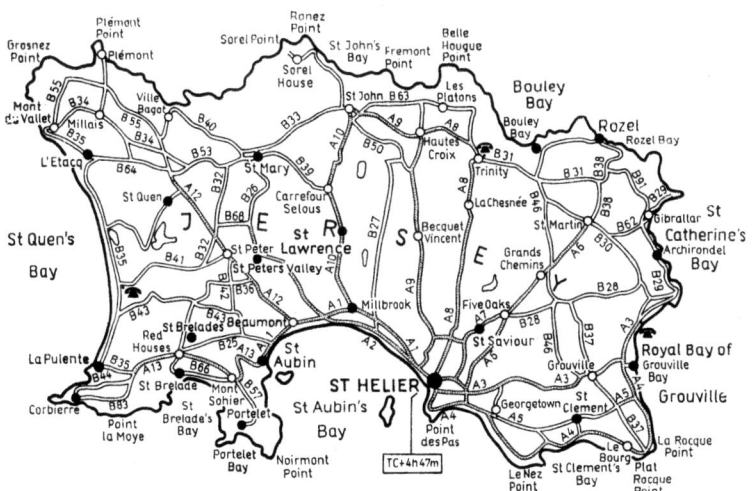

TEST
32

Typical test types for special professions 50

TEST **Notes – visual testing charts I**

33 This consists of different sizes of notes used in note print (i. e. pieces of printed music). In (a) the distance between the lowest and uppermost line of notes is 7.5 mm, in (b) 7 mm, in (c) 6.5 mm, in (d) 6 mm, in (e) 5.5 mm, in (f) 5 mm, in (g) 4.5 mm, in (h) 4 mm, and in (i) 3.5 mm. They are used according to their intended purpose, e. g. (b) and (c) for orchestra instruments, keyboard-instruments and chamber music, (d) for guitar, (e) and (f) for vocal and choir music as well as orchestral scores for conductors, (g) for the orienting survey of notes, (h) and (i) for study scores. The note tests should be used at the specific distance for playing the respective instruments.

TEST **Notes – visual testing charts II**

34 This presents the three most usual sizes of note.

Typical test types for special professions

TEST 33

Typical test types for special professions

TEST 34

a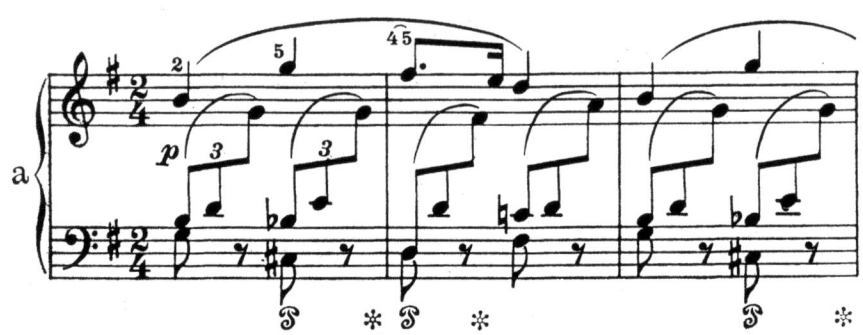

b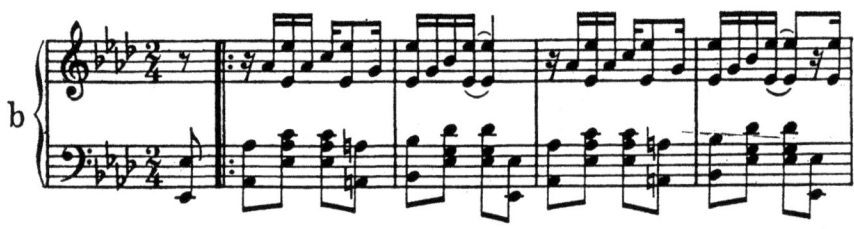

c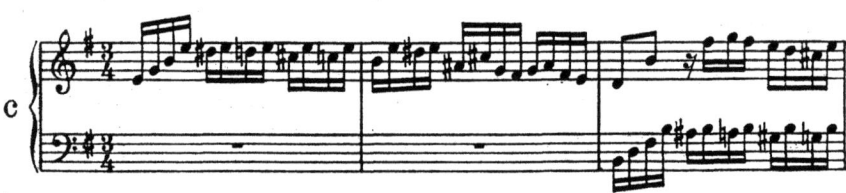

Part of the telephone directory

TEST 35

LONDON S–Z

Ziegler C.A.O.L,Sclr, 4 Bedford Rw WC1	01-242 7363
Ziegler D, 10 Kemplay Rd NW3	01-435 6064
Ziegler E.A, 10 Paultons St SW3	01-352 6246
Ziegler G, 46 Hidaburn Ct,Aldrington Rd SW16	01-769 7460
Ziegler G.A, 69 Peel St W8	01-229 3271
Ziegler H.J, 6 Sherriff Ct,Sherriff Rd NW6	01-625 5562
Ziegler J.R, 7 St. Lukes St SW3	01-352 1663
Ziegler K.A, 62 Addison Rd W14	01-602 5350
Ziegler M, 64 Ridgway Pl SW19	01-946 5437
Ziegler M.L, 24 Ferry Rd SW13	01-748 6763

Newspaper types

TEST 36

BBC-1: 6.0 Ceefax am. 6.30 Breakfast Time. 9.0 The Best of Collecting Now. 9.30 Pages from Ceefax. 10.30 Play School. 10.55 Pages from Ceefax. 12.30 News. 1.0 Pebble Mill at One. 1.45 King Rollo. 1.50 Bric-a-Brac. 2.0 The Afternoon Show. 2.40 Truck Drivin' Man. 3.25 Arthur Negus Enjoys. 3.50 Magic Roundabout. 3.55 Play School. 4.20 Laurel and

POCONOS FORECLOSURE
Poconos-near Camelback Ski area. Finance co. must sell foreclosure lot over 1/3 acr in estate setting. Pay off $8000 unpaid bal.cn this $14,000 lot, no money down,payment $154 per mo. Lake, golf course, swim & tennis ct & paved rds. Prop is ready to build on or hold for investment. Minutes to ski area & Caesar's resort properties (is

TIME SHARE FORECLOSURES
Developer's Closeouts & Resales.

Vacation Financial Corp is pleased to offer one of the best buys in real estate history. We have acquired 500 weeks in hospitality award winning resort. Purchase of one of these RCI deeded weeks will facilitate vacation accommodations in 900 resorts world wide.

Everyday tests / Tests for special purposes 54

TEST 37   Tickets

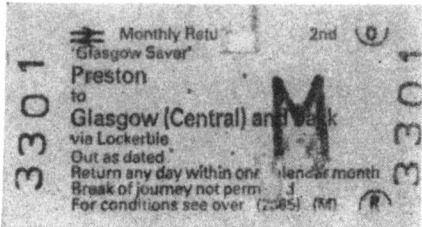

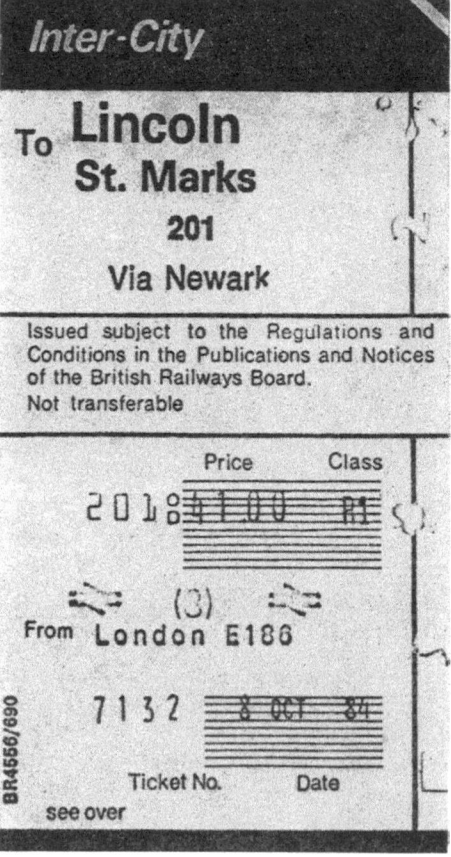

Time-table

TEST **38**

			☒	☒		☒	☒		☒	☒
London Waterloo ⊖	147	d	09 12	..	09 28	09 42	..	09 58	10 12	..
Clapham Junction	147	d	09 19	..	09 35	09 49	..	10 05	10 19	..
Putney	147	d	09 23	..	..	09 53	..	..	10 23	..
Richmond (Surrey) ⊖	147	d	09 29	..	09 44	09 59	..	10 14	10 29	..
Twickenham	147	d	09 36	..	..	10 02	..	..	10 32	..
Whitton	147	d	09 39	..	..	10 05	..	..	10 35	..
Feltham		d	09 43	..	09 51	10 09	..	10 21	10 39	..
Ashford (Surrey)		d	09 47	..	..	10 13	..	..	10 43	..
Staines		d	09 52	09 54	09 57	10 16	10 22	10 27	10 46	10 52

Visual testing charts for the screen reading device

(positive and negative picture reproduction)

TEST **39**

The screen reading device assists reading and writing in patients with a high degree of vision impairment, particularly, those with macula and tapetoretinal degeneration, atrophy of the optic nerve, high degree myopia and amblyopia. With the more sophisticated electronic devices a magnification to 45-fold is possible, after switching to an additional electronic magnifying glass even to 60-fold. Vision should be between 0.1 and 0.01 and the visual field should at least have a size of 2° in order to obtain reading ability for newspaper print. Often a practice attempt at the screen reading device is necessary.

The tests 39 and 40 contain words in newspaper types in a 10-fold and 20-fold magnification, respectively, with positive and negative reproduction.

TEST **40**

Tests for special purposes

TEST 39

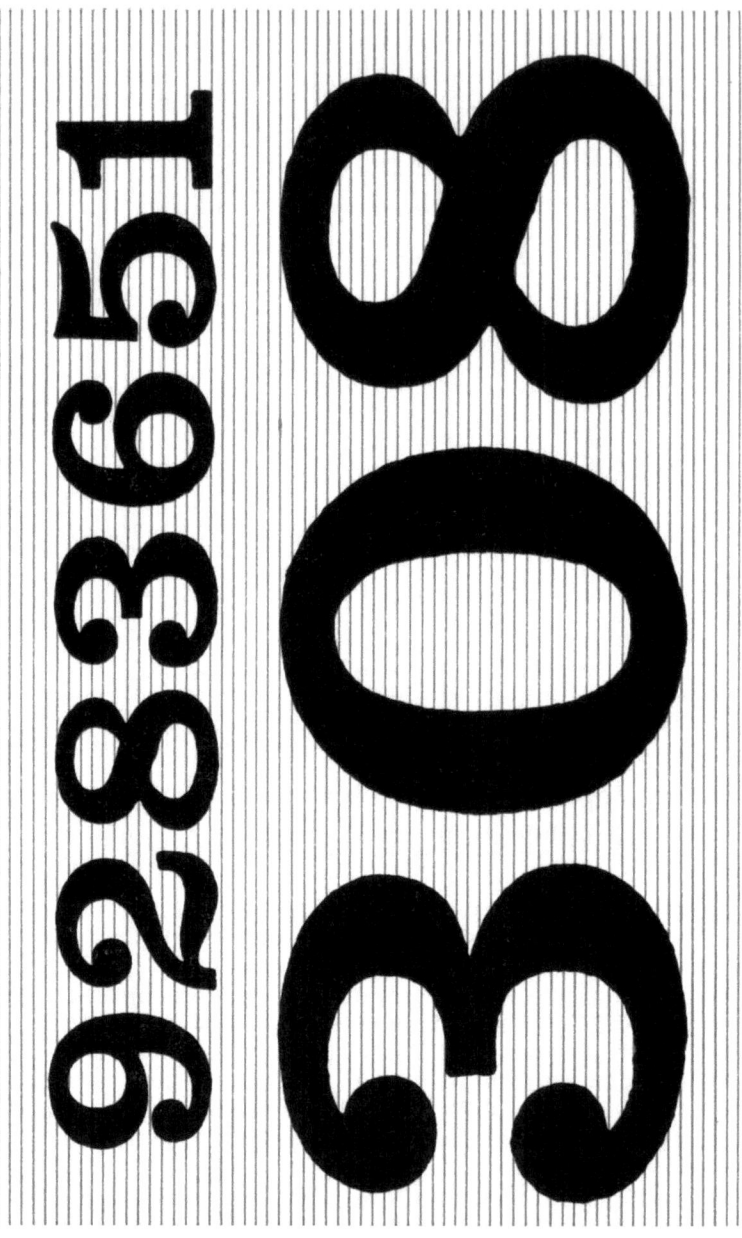

Tests for special purpose

**TEST
40**

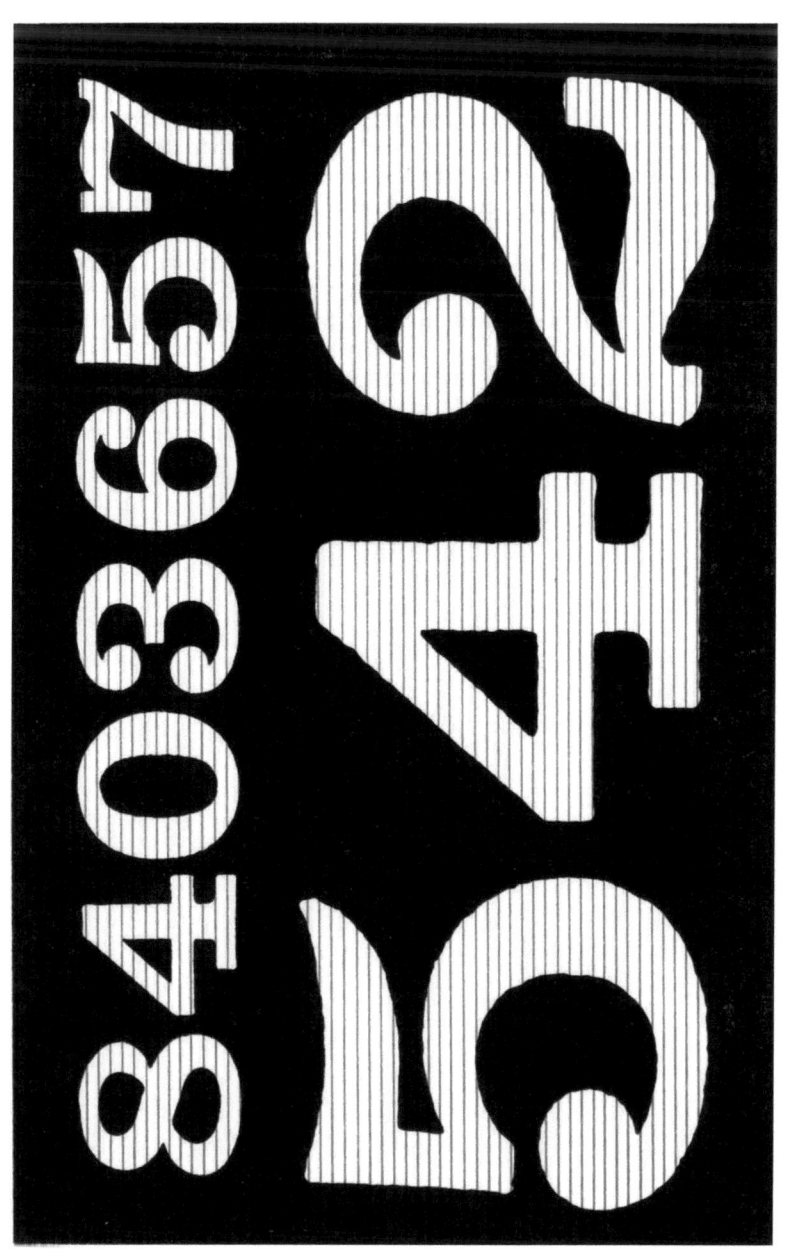

Tests for special purposes	58

TEST 41 **Anaglyph**

Through one of the enclosed red-blue-spectacles and through the red-green-spectacle of the Worth- or TNO-tests, respectively, the diagram can be plastically (stereoscopically) recognized as a relief (red in front of the left eye).

Above and below mountains are seen, in the centre a valley. If the test or the holder is turned by 180°, then the mountains represent themselves as valleys and vice versa. By means of these four possibilities of demonstration a dissimulation can effectively be encountered.

The test must not be performed tilted. The distance of observation shall be about 33 cm. With a visual acuity of less than 5/20 the test fails, since several points of details are no longer perceived. The clear recognition of the stereo-effects in the relief reliably proves the existence of stereo-vision.

Due to the stereo-retardation in haploscopic stereo-patterns an observation time of several seconds is required in order to obtain a stereoscopic impression.

Tests for special purposes

**TEST
41**

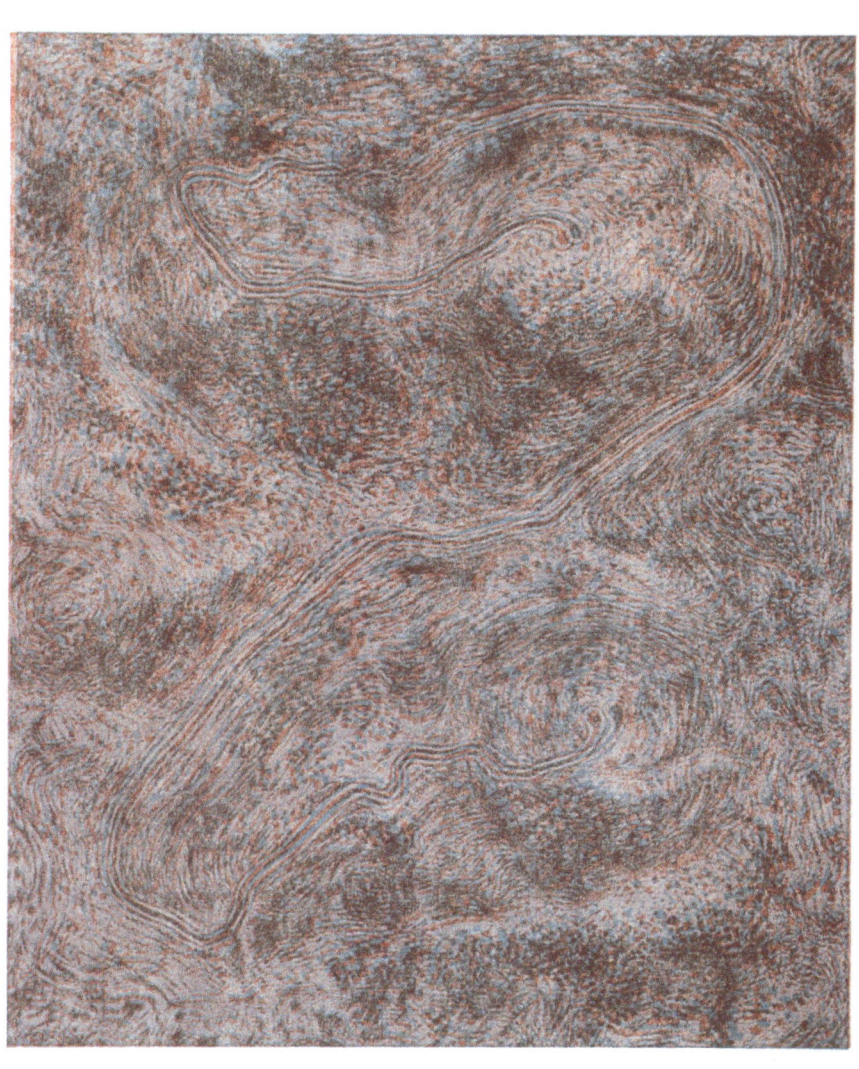

Tests for special purposes

TEST 42

Examination of the central visual field

Not infrequently central or paracentral scotomas are the cause of a reduced professional visual power. Central scotomas and central metamorphopsias can be established by means of the grid of test 42. The patient looks with one eye into the centre of the test and states which lines of the grid he does not perceive or perceives with contortion, and draws the result on a chequered sheet of paper of the same size.

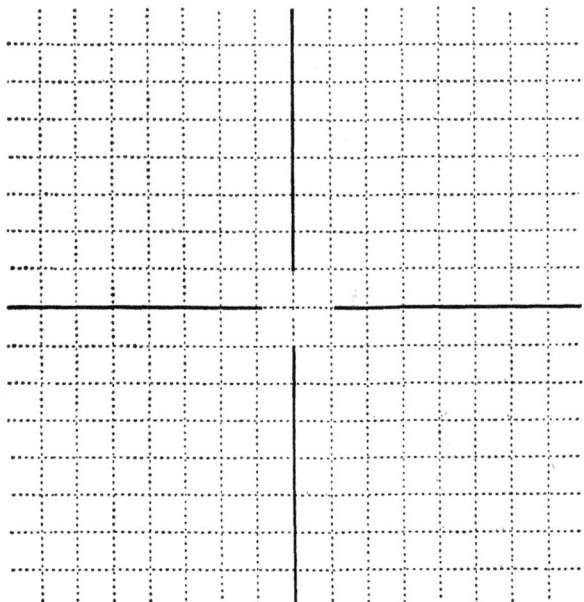

Tests for special purposes

TEST 43

Measurement of short-distance exo- and esophoria

For testing the short-distance exo- and esophoria (distance 30 cm) a prismatic glass with 6 prdpt is put before the left eye (basis above). Looking through the red-blue-spectacles (red before the left eye), the patient sees the scale double. The red arrow put vertically indicates the exophoria (left side) or the esophoria (right side) at the scale appearing below.

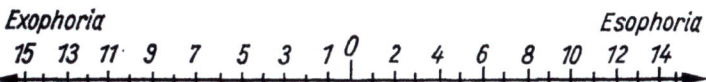

TEST 44 Braille

Patients who become to a great extent amblyope or blind not infrequently ask for the opportunity to learn braille.
The test can demonstrate braille to the patient with the help of the braille alphabet as well as a series of numbers.

TEST 45 Relief demonstrations for blind

Literature

Amsler, M.: Zur Frühdiagnose und Frühbehandlung von Makulaerkrankungen. Klin. Mbl. Augenheilk. **122**, 385-388 (1953)

Barth, Ch., und M. Sachsenweger: Die Eignung von Anaglyphenreliefs zur Prüfung des stereoskopischen Sehens. Z. Verkehrsmed. u. Grenzgeb. 28, 5 (1981)

Blankenagel, A., und W. Jaeger: Das Fernsehlesegerät für hochgradig Sehbehinderte. Klin. Mbl. Augenheilk. **163**, 376-380 (1973)

Sachsenweger, M.: Ein neuer Siebtest zur Sehschärfenprüfung bei Vorschulkindern. Augenoptik **94**, 164-166 (1977)

Sachsenweger, M.: Nahsehproben mit Notenschrift. Folia ophthal. **6**, 60-64 (1981)

Sachsenweger, M.: Verwendung des typographischen Maßsystems für Leseproben. Folia ophthal. 9, 183–186 (1984)

Schober, H.: Das Sehen, Bd. 2. Fachbuchverlag, Leipzig 1954, 287-303

Schober, H.: Prüfung der Sehfunktionen. In: W. Straub: Die ophthalmologischen Untersuchungsmethoden, Bd. 2. F. Enke, Stuttgart 1976, Tab. 2

M. Sachsenweger: Near Visual Acuity Tests and professional vision testing charts

Additional test type for everyday use

N. 3 / V = 1.0

The Gulf Stream comes from the Gulf of Mexico and brings warm water to the coasts of Western Europe. – 7 35 809 2413 37689 129456 2340291 85762401 304829812 1239081382 15297461074

N. 4 / V = 0.75

The Sahara in North Africa, the largest desert of the world, comprises about 7 to 9 million square kilometres. – 2 80 167 9684 8713 20934 90184

N. 5 / V = 0.6

Lake Victoria, the largest lake of Africa, is located 1134 m above sea-level. – 2 73 908 6518 24971 682043 8963013

N. 6 / V = 0.5

The Andes extend along the west coast of the South American continent. – 5 82 035 8149 24701 369

N. 7 / V = 0.43

The Ural Mountains and the River Ural form the boundary between Europe and Asia.

N. 8 / V = 0.38

On Iceland there are numerous active volcanos. – 9 72 560 3152 69052 897130

N. 9 / V = 0.33

Australia is considered to be the smallest continent. – 7 42 069 8726

N. 10 / V = 0.3

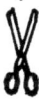
The Indian Ocean is the smallest of the three oceans. – 7 35

N. 11 / V = 0.27

The Volga is considered to be the longest and most copiously flowing river of Europe. − 3 85 018 6427 5902413

N. 12 / V = 0.25

Berne is the capital of Switzerland. − 7 45 190 682

N. 14 / V = 0.21

Sicily is in the Mediterranean Sea. − 9 26 017

N. 16 / V = 0.19

Frankfurt-on-Main. − 7 25 903 8761359

N. 18 / V = 0.17

The Highlands of Scotland. − 0 67

N. 20 / V = 0.15

Vienna on the Danube. − 2 14

N. 24 / V = 0.13

Great Britain. − 5 49 823

N. 28 / V = 0.11

Pacific Ocean. − 3 286

Test 44

BRAILLE

a	b	c	d	e	f	g	h	i	j	k	l	m
n	o	p	q	r	s	t	u	v	w	x	y	z
1	2	3	4	5	6	7	8	9	0			

Verlag: Deutsche Zentralbücherei für Blinde zu Leipzig

TEST 45

□ ⠋⠊⠛⠂ ⠁⠆ △ ⠙⠗⠊⠂ ⠚⠶⠛⠄

▭ ⠗⠂⠽⠂ ⠚⠶⠛⠄ ○ ⠉⠑⠗⠉⠄

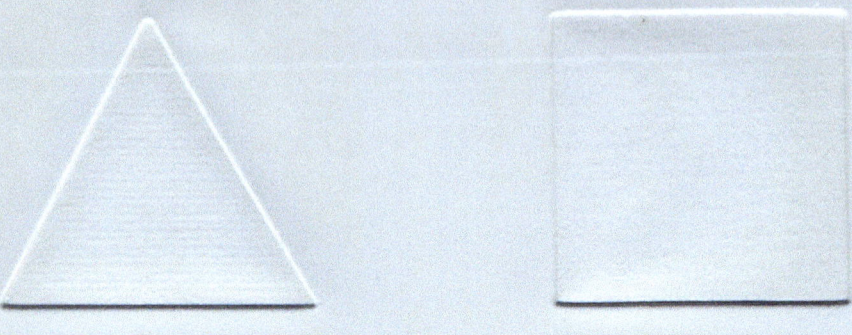

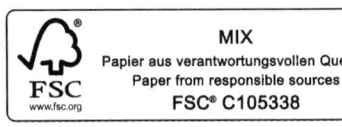

If you have any concerns about our products,
you can contact us on
ProductSafety@springernature.com

In case Publisher is established outside the EU,
the EU authorized representative is:
**Springer Nature Customer Service Center GmbH
Europaplatz 3, 69115 Heidelberg, Germany**

Printed by Libri Plureos GmbH
in Hamburg, Germany